Yoga as we know it!

Aisosa Philip Morgan.

Some Yoga poses

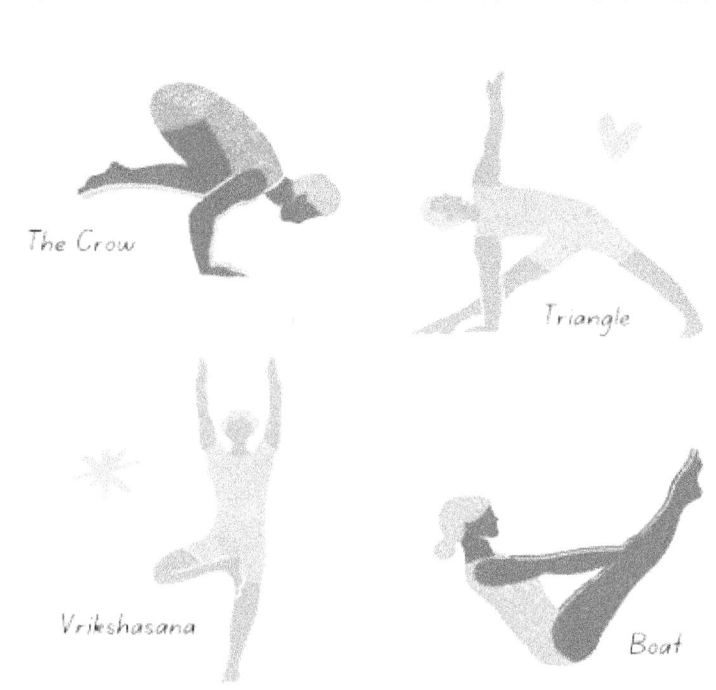

The Crow
Triangle
Vrikshasana
Boat

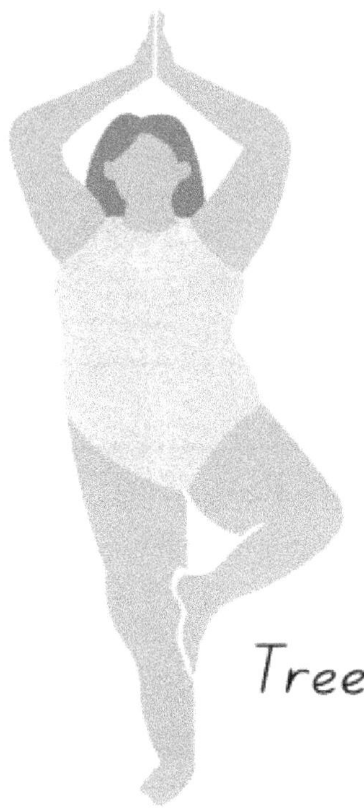

A note from the author

Hey! Thanks for reading in advance.I know there are millions of yoga books out there but you chose to read mine so it's appreciated. If you are a beginner and you have never tried yoga,i hope that this book will help you.The title of this book is somewhat of a delightful, zen-like joke because the journey of yoga is one that is constantly an introduction. Yoga never ends; it is an ongoing practice of self-discovery and recharging your body for optimum health.

With that stated, it's perfectly ok to refer to something as an introduction to yoga for strictly pragmatic reasons, and perhaps this book has been a nice eye-opener for you.

CH 1

What do we mean by Yoga?

Yoga is a collection of physical, mental, and spiritual exercises that have their roots in ancient India. They are meant to calm the mind and recognize a detached witness awareness that is unaffected by the mind and everyday suffering.It is an age-old technique that calls for certain physical postures, mental focus, and deep breathing.

Regular yoga practice can enhance stamina, power, serenity, flexibility, and general wellbeing.Over 5,000 years ago in northern India, yoga first appeared.

When one of India's well-known gurus, Swami Vivekananda, was welcomed at the World Fair in Chicago in 1893, the practice of yoga first reached the west. He is now recognized for having spurred interest in yoga in the West.

Yoga literally translates to "to yoke, bind, unite, or direct one's attention" from the Sanskrit word Yug. In addition, yoga may allude to ideas like fusion, union, and discipline.

Yoga is referred to as a "unitive discipline" in the sacred texts of Hinduism, an ancestor of world religions with roots in India. According to academics Georg Feuerstein and Stephan Bodian in their book Living Yoga, this discipline promotes inner and exterior union, harmony, and joy.

Yoga is not a form of exercise. Yoga does, in fact, contain a lot of postures, particularly in hatha yoga, but these are merely there to help people connect with their inner feelings.

Contrary to what many people are encouraged to believe, yoga is not a religion or a method of meditation. The process of bringing ourselves into the spiritual world includes more than just meditation.

CH 2

Physical Health and Yoga.

Yoga does not distinguish between the body and the mind, and western psychology has come to the same conclusion for a very long time (the link between mental health and physical health, and vice versa).

Please don't panic; you've come to the correct place if you've come to this book hoping to understand yoga as a way to assist your body heal or improve.

In fact, yoga is a procedure that involves unblocking energy and tension in the body and assisting in maximizing the function of the muscles, tendons, joints, ligaments, and all other parts.

According to yoga, stiffness and lack of mobility only occur when the body is sick or out of alignment. Humans are, by nature, best suited to being flexible and agile.

In order to improve their physical health, many people have found themselves in yoga classes or at home on a yoga mat watching yoga videos or DVDs. You could be one of them. If so, you can either continue reading or put the book down right now. I won't push you to do anything.

Physical Benefits of Yoga include

stretched-out joints and a wider range of motion

joint and muscle discomfort is lessened

improved immunity

improved lung function and better respiratory quality

an accelerated metabolism (which can result in weight loss!)

increased sleep standards (especially due to improved breathing and a more oxygenated body)

Yoga has always aided in promoting the body's flexibility and in lubricating the joints, ligaments, and tendons. This is because some yoga practices call for certain postures to be mastered. Yoga helps the body detox by improving blood flow to numerous organs. It aids in toning and energizing muscles that have become weak and flabby.

Please remember that while yoga is frequently addressed in terms of its mental approach, this technique also has definite and established physical advantages.

Therefore, yoga is as viable a choice for you as it is for the stressed-out corporate executive who needs to find a method of coping with the chaos of your busy life,or weight reduction or the capacity to shovel snow without having your back suffer for days in winter is your aim.

CH 3

Why is yoga good for you?

Yoga through meditation is an incredibly effective way to create harmony and makes the mind and body more in tune. How frequently do we find that the conflicts and confusions in our minds make it difficult for us to carry out our tasks effectively and satisfactorily?

The most likely culprit affecting every aspect of our endocrine, hormonal, and emotional systems is stress. And these issues can be resolved with the assistance of yoga.

Yoga and its purifying techniques have successfully treated many diseases on a physical level.

Complete body cleansing is provided by yoga. Yoga ensures the best blood supply to various body areas by gently stretching the muscles and joints and massaging the various organs. This aids in eliminating toxins from every crevice of your body and supplying nourishment all the way to the end. As a result, there are advantages like postponed aging, vigor, and a fantastic love for life.

Yoga is a fantastic exercise for building muscle. Repetitive stimulation causes flaccid and weak muscles to burn more fat and tighten up.

The ability to do incredible physical feats through the power of the mind is now a well-known fact, demonstrating the link between the mind and body beyond a shadow of a doubt.

Yoga and meditation actually work together to achieve the same objective of obtaining mind, body, and spirit unification, which can result in a feeling of eternal happiness that you can only have through practicing yoga.

Through detachment, yoga's meditation techniques assist in establishing emotional balance.

This in turn fosters a fantastic sense of calmness and optimism, both of which have a profoundly favorable impact on one's physical well-being.

The mind-body connection is the main focus of yoga. Three things help to create this balance of the mind and body:

Postures (asanas)
> proper breathing techniques (pranayama)
> Meditation

The integrated practices of asanas, breathing, and meditation provide inspiration and direction for both the mind and the body. Our bodies become more vulnerable to toxins and poisons as we become older (yogis believe that aging is an artificial phenomenon) (caused by environmental and poor dietary factors).

Yoga guides us through a purification process that makes our bodies work together like a well-oiled machine.

These three principles must be balanced in order to reap the rewards of yoga. And what exactly are these advantages? These advantages consist of:
> a state of equilibrium in the body's neurological system
> Pulse rate dropping
> blood pressure and respiratory rates
> vascular effectiveness
> stabilized gastrointestinal system
> lengthened breath-holding
> enhanced dexterity abilities.
> enhanced balance
> more accurate depth perception

CH 4

Mental and psychological advantages of yoga

People frequently bring out the physiological advantages of yoga, such as improved strength, flexibility, and relaxation, while discussing the practice.

The advantages of a yoga practice for the mind, body, and brain are not discussed enough, though. Yoga has been demonstrated to be beneficial in lowering anxiety and sadness as well as some forms of Post-Traumatic Stress Disorder, according to a review published in Harvard Mental Health in 2009. Additionally, a number of new research indicate that yoga may support stronger social ties, stress reduction, and sleeplessness relief.

Some of the psychological advantages of regular yoga practice include:

Relaxation: A key component of yoga is learning how to breathe deeply from the abdomen, which has been shown to lower blood levels of the stress hormone cortisol. Yoga can so aid in your relaxation and stress reduction, allowing you to think more clearly.

Help to relax the mind: Paying attention to your breathing and bodily movements might help you reduce mental clutter and gain insight about what is really bothering you.

Increasing your awareness of your physical self might sometimes help you become more in touch with your emotions by bringing them to the surface.

Principles of mindfulness: Worries are either future- or past-focused. Yoga helps us to fully concentrate on the present moment and to be present in it. By putting our attention on the here and now and asking ourselves, "What is within my power and control at this moment?" we can benefit from practicing mindfulness in our daily lives.

Distress Patience: Yoga principles encourage us to lean into the discomfort, whether it's tolerating the heat in a Bikram yoga class or holding a challenging position. Yoga practice teaches us to not be afraid of suffering and gives us self-assurance that we can handle the pain by breathing, keeping our balance, and being present in the moment.

As was already mentioned, there are a number of psychological advantages to practicing yoga, and this is actually a fairly popular reason why individuals first start doing it. An better capacity to regulate stress may be the psychological advantage of yoga that is emphasized the most. Yoga reduces a person's levels of worry, despair, and lethargy, allowing them to concentrate on what is spiritually and ultimately significant finding balance and happiness.

Please keep in mind that yoga cannot guarantee that anyone will experience these benefits immediately. At most, yoga is the light that reveals how disorganized your basement actually is. Once the light is turned on, cleaning up is considerably simpler, more effective, and less time-consuming.

CH 5

Emotional benefits of Yoga

Yoga has also been praised for its unique capacity to aid individuals in getting rid of their internal animosity and bitterness. The doorway to self actualization and self acceptance opens as a result of eradicating these harmful emotions.

Emotions frequently result from our internal reaction to anything external to us. Being aware of our thoughts and feelings is therefore one of the emotional advantages of yoga. When our thoughts are evoking an unwelcome emotional reaction, we can tell.

For instance, we might get angry frequently. We will first realize that rage is our characteristic emotion if we practice yoga and develop mindfulness. The predisposition to believe individuals are cruel or out to get us may then become apparent to us. Such a link enables us to comprehend our anger, which frequently causes it to subside.

Yoga has emotional advantages that affect both the body and the mind. This is only one of the many benefits of yoga. It has the power to alter both our thoughts and feelings.

First, yoga can help us alter how we physically perceive emotions. If we experience a lot of anxiety, we can try a relaxing exercise like restorative or gentle yoga. We can also practice breathing techniques and meditation to calm down or manage our rage.

When we're depressed, we could experience excessive exhaustion or a lack of energy. An energized vinyasa practice or a breathing technique like "breath of fire" may be helpful in that situation.

Yoga also affects mental wellbeing in various ways. As previously noted, mindfulness meditation can assist us in becoming more conscious of our emotions and the relationship between our ideas and feelings. This awareness frequently has the unexpected result of lessening the impact of unpleasant feelings.

Additionally, research indicates that yoga may alter brain chemistry. In particular, it might aid in raising levels of serotonin, a chemical that controls mood. Regular yoga practice can also aid in increasing endorphins, which are linked to a sense of general wellbeing.

Yoga's capacity to foster joyful emotions is one of its additional emotional advantages. When we practice yoga, we not only feel better physically, but we frequently gain the emotional advantage of meaningfully connecting with others who share our interests.

Dedicated yogis are frequently pleasantly surprised by the emotional advantages of yoga. Many people who start a yoga practice for physical fitness, stress relief, or spiritual enlightenment end up getting more than they bargained for. They gradually experience less grief, rage, and terror as well.

Do you struggle to control your emotions? Consider rolling out your yoga mat right now.

yoga can also be beneficial in the reduction of pain. Being aware of the beneficial relationship between yoga and pain management could be extremely helpful given that everyone experiences pain and chronic pain at some time.

CH 6

Various Forms of Yoga

Six primary varieties of yoga are noted by yogic researchers Feuerstein and Bodian. They are, in no particular order:

1.Hatha yoga: Hatha yoga is a 5000-year-old system that was utilized to improve overall well-being of the body, mind, and soul. Asanas, which are stretches, are incorporated into the practice of Hatha Yoga. It incorporates breathing exercises and mental focus.

Hatha Yoga is practiced in the Lotus pose from the Asanas.

The aim of practicing Hatha Yoga is identical to that of practicing other forms of Yoga. It seeks to unite the tranquil spirit of the universe with the human spirit. The individual doing yoga improves their spiritual, mental, physical, and emotional health and aspect with this practice.

By practicing Hatha Yoga, you may maintain world peace and a peaceful environment.

Hatha Yoga's primary goal is to have the body ready to submit so that the spirit can take in and complete its task. The spirit is in charge of uplifting and illuminating. When the spirit is awakened, the mind is at ease and free from tension and suffering. The body also does.

Too many people are perplexed since they do not comprehend that your spirit cannot successfully complete the mission if your body is unhealthy and inadequate. So if your spirit is weak, Hatha Yoga is the ideal practice to use.

Hatha yoga will support you in getting your body moving and improving to a point where the spirit can function properly. For your intellect to be able to keep up with good focus, your spirit and body must react favorably.

Hatha Yoga is typically the first type of yoga that people think of when they hear the phrase. The most widely practiced kind of yoga is Hatha. In actuality, Hatha Yoga is where other forms of yoga like Kundalini, Ashtanga, Bikram, and Power Yoga got their start.

The greatest benefit of Hatha yoga is that it enables you to discover for yourself that you possess a divine light. In addition to enlightening you, it can also make you stronger, more at ease, and more adaptable.

Hatha yoga involves physical activity that opens energy pathways to allow the flow of spiritual energy. If the mind, body, and spirit are in harmony and in good operating order, this will be possible. The most crucial thing to remember is to keep your body healthy. When your body is compromised, it also affects your mind and spirit.

You can manage stress and reduce some pain and tension when you practice Hatha Yoga. You occasionally need to unwind because working so hard can leave you drained and worn out. The best treatment to relieve the pain and tension is Hatha Yoga.

2.Yoga raja:Raja Yoga is regarded as the "royal route" to bringing the body and mind into harmony, just like classical yoga is. Raja yoga, which seeks enlightenment via direct control and mastery of the mind, is regarded by some as a particularly challenging style of yoga.

Raja yoga is best suited for those who prefer meditation and have good attention spans. This branch of yoga contains eight limbs:

moral restraint

posture, restriction, breathing control, sensory inhibition, concentration

meditation

ecstasy

3.Karma yoga:Karma yoga calls for unselfish deeds. The word "karma" itself denotes activity, including all deeds committed by a person from the moment of his birth till his passing. Karma is the road to doing the right thing, which is most important. Karma yoga therefore involves letting up of the ego in order to serve God and humanity.

The Bhagavad Vita, sometimes affectionately referred to as "the New Testament of Hinduism," is the source of karma yoga. Karma Yoga is built on the principle of serving God by serving others.

4.Bhakti yoga: Bhakti yoga is viewed as heavenly love. Swami Nikhilananda and Sri Ramakrishna Math assert that love functions on three levels as an attractive force:

Material\Human\Spiritual

These two gurus go on to say that love is a creative force that drives us to pursue happiness and immortality.

5.Jnana yoga:The way to wisdom is through jnana yoga. According to Graham Ledgerwood, jnana entails "emptying out" one's mind and spirit of illusions in order to become attuned to truth and letting go of all ideas and feelings up until one is transformed and enlightened.

One of the four basic routes that leads directly to self-realization is jnana yoga (philosophy of advaita vedanda).

The practice of jnana yoga allows the student to encounter God by overcoming ignorance's barriers.

In Jnana yoga, where the practitioner or student recognizes himself as distinct from the elements of his surroundings, ideas like discernment and discrimination are highly valued. Jnana Yoga likewise adheres to the "Neti-Neti" idea. Literally, it means "not this, not this," because when things are taken away, all that is left is you.

6.Tantra yoga:Some people believe that of all the yoga branches, tantric yoga is the most oriental. It is frequently believed to just involve sexual practices. It is a route to self-transcendence by ritual means, one of which is simply consecrated sexuality, and it involves more than just having sex. After a certain point, some tantric schools even suggest leading a celibate existence.

Tantra means "expanding" in Sanskrit. A Tantra practitioner raises all levels of consciousness in order to approach the Supreme Reality. Tantra yoga seeks to arouse a person's male and female sides in order to cause a spiritual awakening.

Tantra yoga focuses more on integrating the body, mind, and spirit, as well as on spiritual healing. In India, there is a long-standing belief that sexuality is a necessary and vital step in achieving a certain level of enlightenment.

Sexual pleasures and wants are not inclined toward or connected to spirituality according to Western religious traditions. There is a thin line between their attitudes and sentiments regarding spirituality and sexuality because of these cultural variances.

Eastern philosophy, on the other hand, lauds and rejoices in the beauty and magnificence of creation.

Later, they created a study or science to comprehend how to make the most of this delightful and healing experience.

In Tantra, energy is recognized as the source of life and is regarded as such.

Additionally, they view the want and power of sexual desire as a powerful and sacred force. A handful of the many workouts and dietary changes are available to aid in the execution of the sexual function. These physical workouts can include holding particular positions, breathing, and contractions.

There are a plethora of advantages to doing these different physical activities. Some of these include enhanced and improved sexual performance as well as improved prostate functioning. An additional advantage is increased sexual endurance during sexual activity.

Exercises come in a variety of forms. There are also psycho-spiritual exercises in addition to physical ones. These exercises can help you learn to meditate on desire and unconditional love. As a result, sexual activities may become less uncomfortable and embarrassing. In addition, there may be less pressure to perform and move.

Giving in totally to your partner or lover's desires is reportedly the most interesting aspect of sexual activity. Expectations may be high, so one must deliver and take action.

One can consider the different ways in which he can appease his beloved through meditation and appropriate exercise. One can deepen their relationship with their partner and also find the fulfillment they have always desired when they are focused and committed to providing their partner what they truly want. When you are concentrating on your sexual performance, there are a few exercises that can be quite helpful.

Yoga is a highly intriguing and traditional method of bringing the body and the mind into harmony, as you now know It has been shown to have positive effects on both physical and emotional wellbeing.

CH 7

Yoga Postures for Novices

If you have never heard of yoga, you will undoubtedly be curious about how the movements are performed and how they appear. Since you are a newbie, you will undoubtedly inquire about the positions that will suit you the best.

The mind and the body are regarded by yogis as two halves of a single entity. This conviction has persisted throughout time without ever failing. Harmony-based self-healing has been extensively practiced through yoga. If you're in the right setting, you can accomplish this.

The positive effects of yoga have persuaded medical professionals that the practice can be helpful for those with conditions that are difficult to treat.

You can practice the yoga poses for beginners and use them on yourself if you suffer from a long-lasting ailment.

You need to have faith in yoga's healing or rejuvenating powers if you want to practice the introductory yoga positions.

Yoga has been practiced for a long time. People continue to get a lot from it today despite the fact that it has been used and practiced for a very long period.

Studies have been conducted to demonstrate the value of yoga in the healing process.

In order to maintain a high level of joint flexibility, it has been demonstrated that the yoga positions for beginners are very effective and useful. Although the yoga positions for beginners are straightforward and uncomplicated, regular practice can gradually develop a healthy lifestyle and bring more.

It's fascinating and fun to execute the yoga positions for beginners. Beginners won't have any trouble keeping up with the exercises because they are so straightforward. The yoga approach has a significant positive impact on our interior glands and organs. It also comprises the bodily sections that receive little stimulation.

Yoga poses help us to strengthen our bodies by concentrating on the thighs, knees, and ankles. Your bones should react right away if you get used to practicing yoga poses every day.

Both sexes supposedly find the buttocks and abdomen to be quite attractive. It is essential for males to maintain a good abdomen of abs. The women find it more enticing as a result.

A lot of women practice in order to get a lot of figure and shape in their bodies, and having a good butt matters to some of them as well.

Sciatica is amazingly relieved by yoga poses. Some pain, like this, is unavoidable. You might not have any back or muscular pain if you practice yoga occasionally, or even consistently.

Here are some tips for maintaining a suitable yoga stance. Simply follow these instructions to thoroughly comprehend yoga positions and be able to perform them correctly.

1.Your heels should be slightly apart while your big toe bases should be in contact. The balls of your feet should also be softly lifted and spread. After that, you must gently lay them on the ground. You can even rock side to side while doing this. You can gradually stop swaying so that you can maintain a standing position with your weight evenly distributed across your feet.

2.The following step is to tighten your thigh muscles, followed by elevating your kneecaps. Don't clench your lower belly while doing it. Lifting the inner ankles will strengthen the internal arches. Next, visualize an energy line running from your inner thighs all the way up to your groins. From there, out through the crown of your head, through the center of your neck, torso, and head. The upper thighs should be slowly rotated inward. Raising the pubis in the direction of the navel while lengthening the tailbone toward the floor.

3.Spread your shoulder blades out transversely, then push them into your back before letting them fall down. Lift your sternum's top straight up toward the ceiling without jarringly pushing your lower front ribs forward. your collarbones should be wider. Alongside the torso, suspend your arms.

4. The base of your chin should be analogous to the floor, your throat should be soft, and your tongue should be broad and plane on the floor of your mouth. Your head should be balanced unwaveringly over the middle of your pelvis. Make your eyes appear kinder.

5.For all of the standing poses in yoga, tadasana is typically the first position. Tansana application is beneficial, particularly when performing the poses. It can be maintained by holding the stance for 30 to 1 minute while breathing normally.

CH 8

Some Yoga poses

1.Seated poses:These yoga positions improve the flexibility of your hips and lower back. Your back gets strengthened as a result. Your knees, groin, ankle, and most significantly your spine gain flexibility as a result. Another benefit is that yoga encourages deep breathing, which makes you feel serene and at peace.

2.Standing poses:One of the essential yoga poses is standing. In order to align your body and your feet, try this stance. Additionally, it helps to maintain and improve healthy posture. It is advantageous since it allows you to stretch and straighten your backbones without even realizing it if you have poor posture. Because your hips and legs are interconnected, standing poses help to strengthen your legs while also increasing their suppleness.

3.Forward bends:This kind aids in both hamstring stretching and lower back strengthening. Your neck, shoulders, and back will feel less tense, and your spine will have more flexibility as a result. This kind of position also promotes calmness.

Back bends are incredibly effective at opening the ribcage, the hips, and even the chest.

This helps to build up and strengthen your arms and shoulders.

It also concurrently improves the elasticity and flexibility of your shoulders. The beautiful thing is that it improves spinal flexibility and helps to release tension from the front of your body up to your hips. You must take good care of your spinal cord because it is one of your body's vital organs.

4.Back bends:You should be aware that the forward bends are difficult because the workout feels good and can help heal some problems. You can use a prop like the strap or the black in this kind of position because it will be really beneficial.

5.Balance poses:Poses requiring balance are quite difficult. Yoga practitioners overexcite themselves when doing balances. This is advantageous because the enjoyment the individual experiences enables him to uplift his spirit and enlighten his soul. Your posture will benefit from having better balance. The spinal cord is lengthened when you have better posture, which helps you avoid falling and getting hurt.

Your capacity to focus on and pay attention to your primary objective can be practiced with balance. However, the highest level of focus should be attained since if your concentration is poor, you can't accomplish this type of pose.

6.Tree pose:You may have heard of this one before.A great way to get started with balancing poses is with tree pose. You can easily exit it if you start to feel like you're about to fall. Avoid extending your hip to the side of your standing leg to generate a counterweight.

Try different foot postures and fix your eyes on a specific area of the floor to find what feels comfortable for you. A low-hanging heel that rests on the ankle, a block, above, or below the knee.

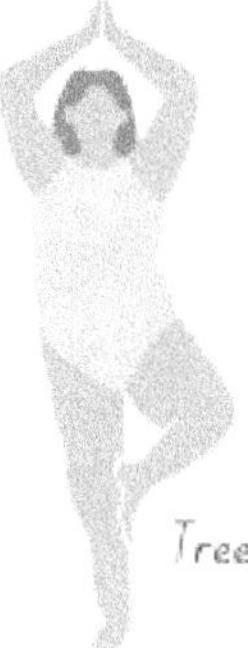

Tree pose

7.Cobra pose:In flow yoga, Cobra is performed several times throughout the vinyasa sequence. While a full cobra with straight arms promotes a deeper backbend, executing low cobras, in which you lift your chest without pressing into your hands, will help you develop more back strength.

As you elevate the sternum, ground into your feet, lengthen through the crown of your head, and expand through your collarbones. Before lifting, it's important to secure your pelvis to the ground.

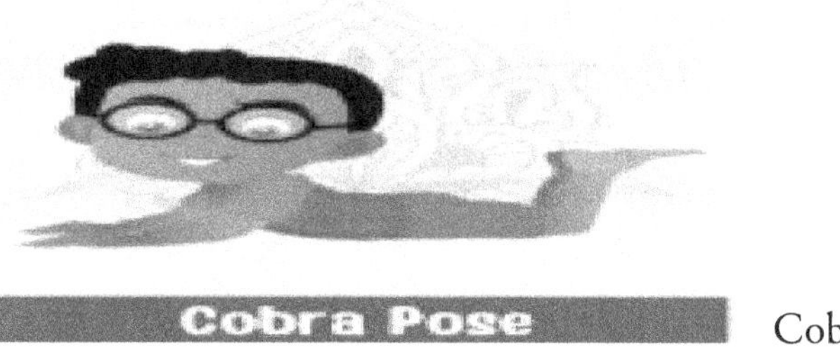

Cobra pose

8.Dancer pose:The lovely balancing stance known as the dancer pose allows you to open your complete front body. Your muscles, attention, and balance are all strengthened by this posture.

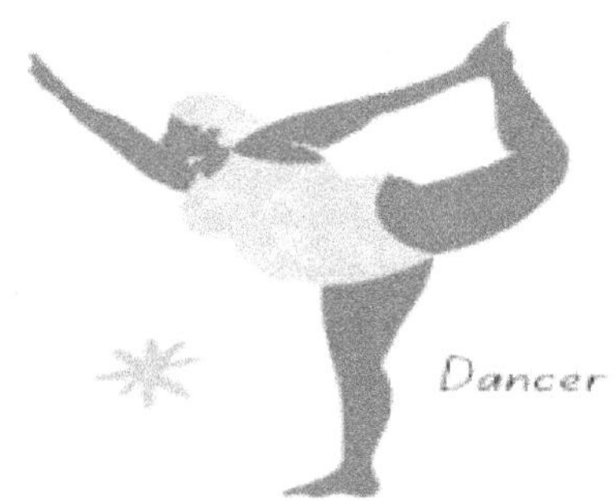

Dancer pose

9.Crow pose:Your legs should rest on your upper arms as you perform the crow pose.

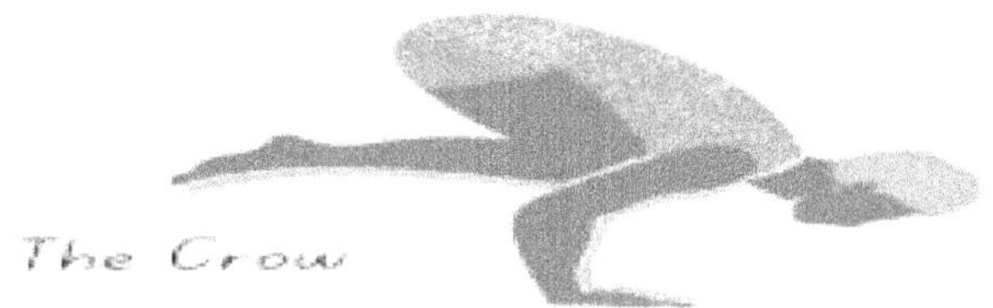

Crow pose

10.Upward dog:Yoga stance known as "Upward-Facing Dog" in the Sun Salutation sequence stretches the upper back, chest, and belly. One of the first backbends you learn in yoga, but it needs to be done correctly to avoid shoulder damage.

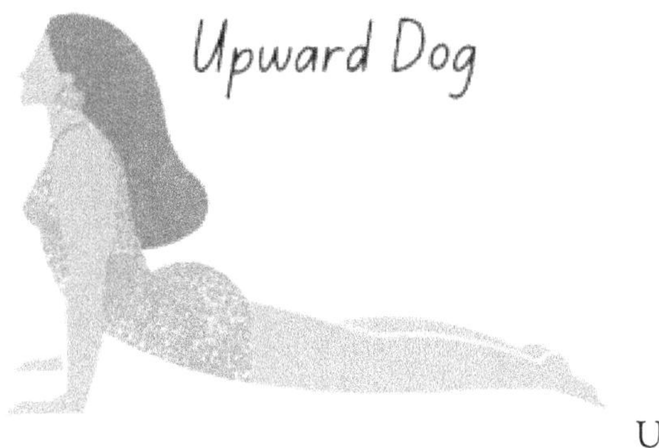

Upward dog

CH 9

Yoga Supplies & Equipment

Pilates Mats or Yoga mats

Start with the well-known yoga mat. Now, as a general rule (with, of course, exceptions), use caution while purchasing the supermarket variety.

A decent yoga mat will have a good grip on the floor, which is crucial if you need to execute challenging poses and movements. They come in a variety of rainbow colors and are normally about 2 feet wide.

You can choose the thickness of yoga mats to meet your needs, from beginner to intermediate. There are several places to buy yoga mats that are well-cushioned. Children can also purchase yoga mats.

Yoga towels

Remember to bring your yoga towel. There are also very absorbent and skid-free towels available in what some stores refer to as "chakra shades."

Gym bags or Yoga bags

Yoga bags have an almost tubular, rectangular appearance and are made to hold your yoga mat, towel, and other equipment.

The majority of goods come with a shoulder strap and are made of various fabrics, with nylon being a popular choice.

Yoga Belts

Many people who practice yoga regularly choose to use yoga straps. They can stretch their limbs and maintain positions for longer thanks to these straps.

yogic music

To improve your meditation, breathe more deeply, and hold certain positions for longer, think about listening to yoga music.

The following are only a few examples of the genres represented: Slow Music for Yoga, Tibetan Sacred Temple Music, Shiva Station, Nectar, Fragrance of the East, etc.

Yoga chants, mantras, audio books, and music for yoga flows are also available.

Yoga attire or clothing

The finest yoga attire is comfortable and allows you to move freely while minimizing distractions and disturbances throughout your practice. For you to avoid irritations, they must feel comfortable on your skin.Yoga attire is a crucial accessory since it helps you get in the mood. Your practice session won't go well if you don't have the right outfit for yoga.

You should expect to perspire excessively throughout a rigorous session. Some people don't really sweat that much, but if you do, you should wear absorbent clothing so that your body's production of sweat is reduced and you feel dry.

No one will reprimand you if you don't have that figure but believe you have the guts. You are the one who must carry your body for as long as you are able to.

The necessities for buying yoga clothing are listed below.

Yoga tops:When selecting a yoga top, the first thing to keep in mind is that it should not fall in your face. When exercising, tops are made to allow you to move freely and focus on your workout. Tee shirts shouldn't be too long or cover the bottom half of your body if you're planning to wear them. Because you can evaluate the alignment of your lower body by looking at your knees and ankles, this is crucial. Most women use sports bras so that when they perform certain exercises, they can be confident that they are being held firmly and that they won't lose them while stretching.

Yoga Pants: Picking out the right pair of yoga pants might be tricky. Some pants' surfaces and textures might not feel comfortable to you. One of the factors to take into account when picking it is the length of the pants. Some pants are so long that your ankles are covered. Wear pants that are below your knees if this is not comfortable for you. You are now free to move about.

Yoga shorts:Yoga shorts are a wonderful option if you practice hot yoga, also referred to as Bikram Yoga. This style of yoga is practiced in a warm room. Your body will release heat if you wear shorts.

Choosing your yoga attire need not be an expensive endeavor. It's crucial that you feel content and at ease on a deep level.

Inspirations and External links

Track yoga
And
https://www.verywellfit.com/essential-yoga-poses-for-beginners-3566747
How to get abs in 4 weeks
https://mybook.to/abs
For the summer(The remaining part at least)
https://mybook.to/xavierreid

About the Author

Author

Self publisher.

His other works include, How to get abs in 4 weeks,Mark of a short and Are eggs good for you.